CW00508562

FACE AGING ZONES

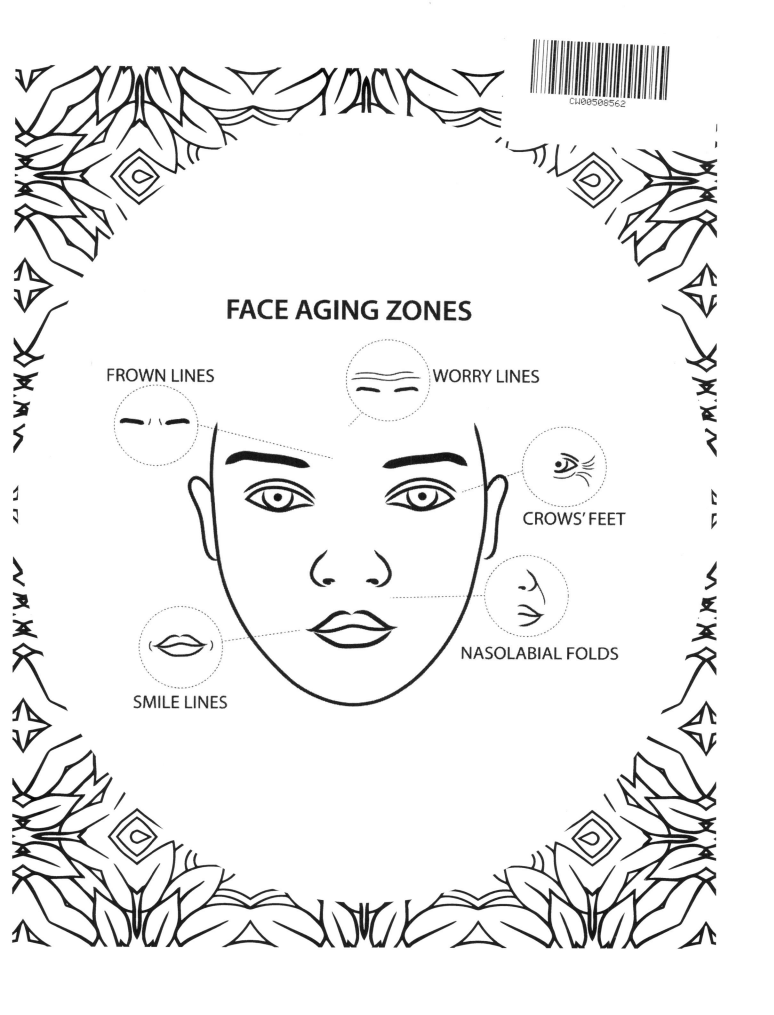

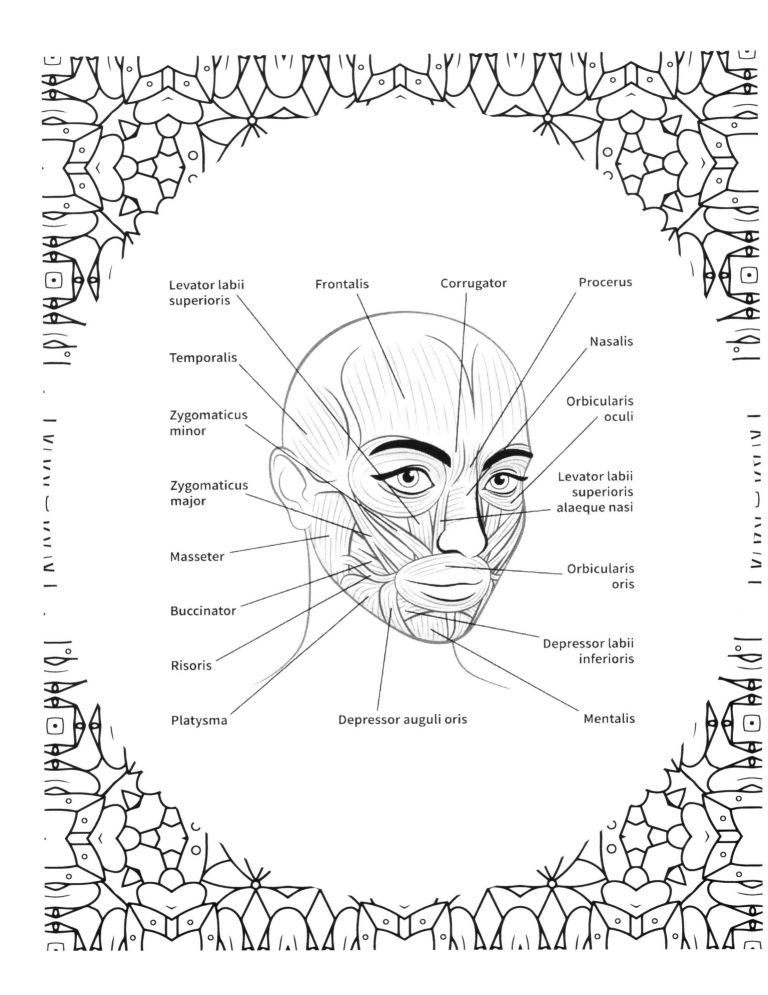

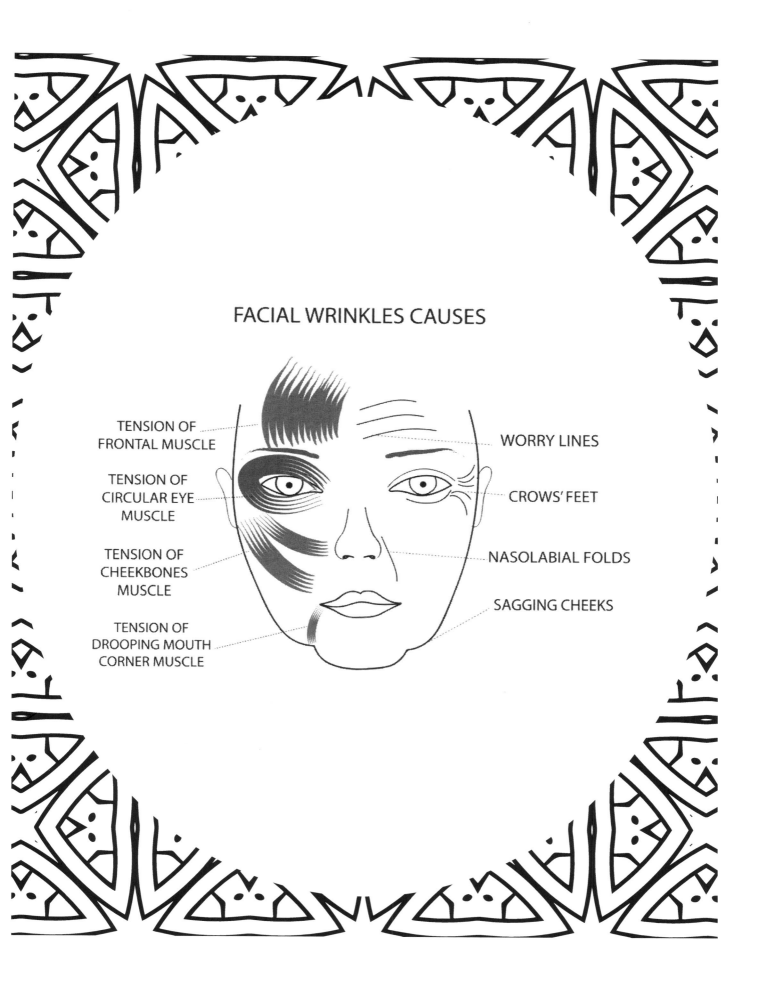

FACIAL WRINKLES CAUSES

TENSION OF
FRONTAL MUSCLE

TENSION OF
CIRCULAR EYE
MUSCLE

TENSION OF
CHEEKBONES
MUSCLE

TENSION OF
DROOPING MOUTH
CORNER MUSCLE

WORRY LINES

CROWS' FEET

NASOLABIAL FOLDS

SAGGING CHEEKS

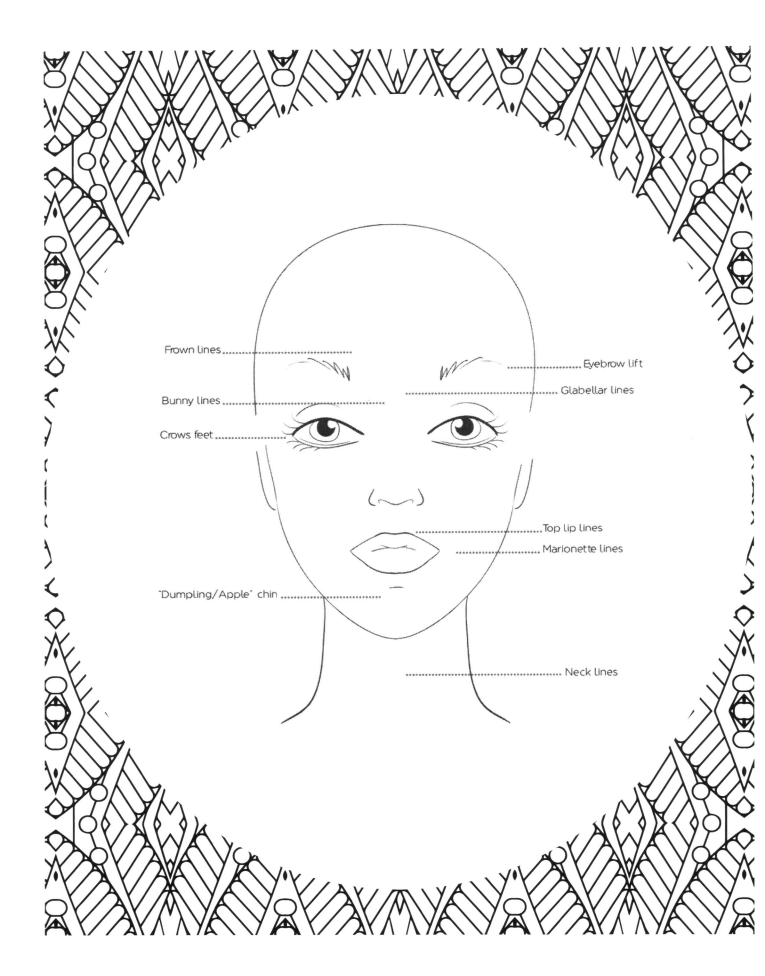

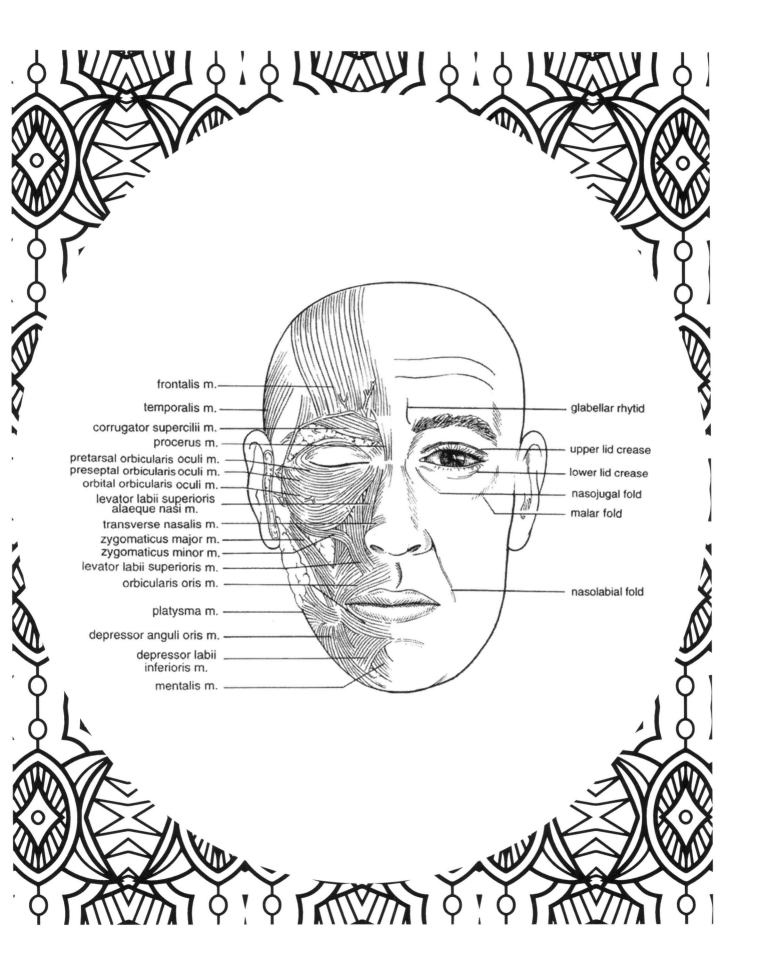

frontalis m.

temporalis m.

corrugator supercilii m.

procerus m.

pretarsal orbicularis oculi m.

preseptal orbicularis oculi m.

orbital orbicularis oculi m.

levator labii superioris
alaeque nasi m.

transverse nasalis m.

zygomaticus major m.

zygomaticus minor m.

levator labii superioris m.

orbicularis oris m.

platysma m.

depressor anguli oris m.

depressor labii
inferioris m.

mentalis m.

glabellar rhytid

upper lid crease

lower lid crease

nasojugal fold

malar fold

nasolabial fold

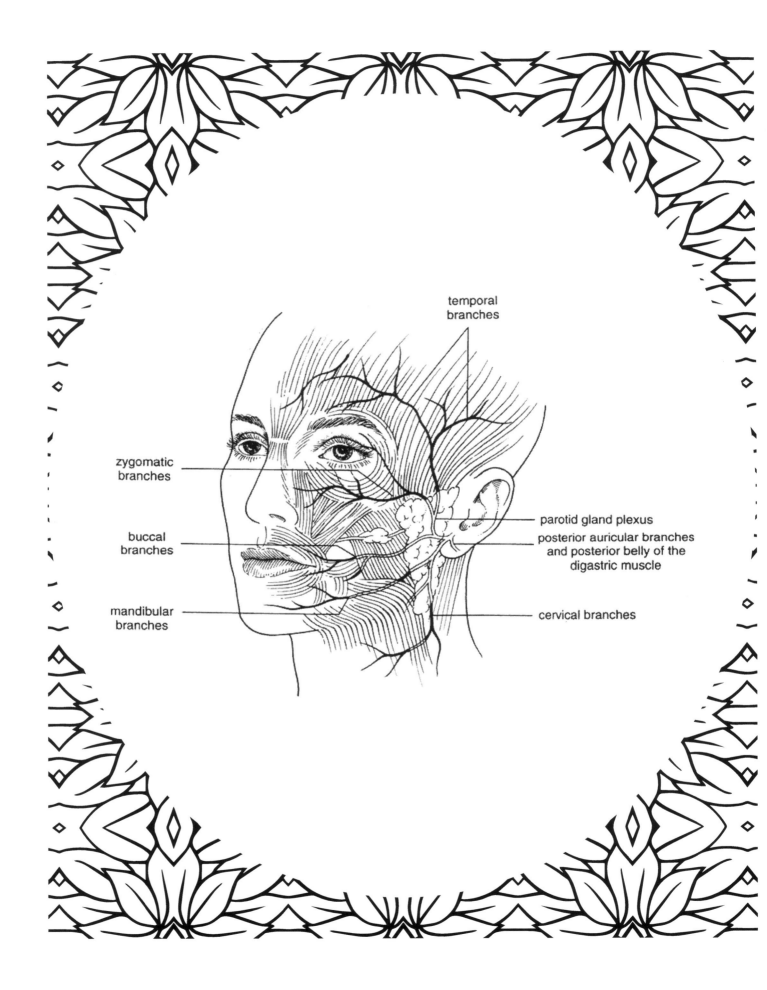

temporal
branches

zygomatic
branches

buccal
branches

mandibular
branches

parotid gland plexus

posterior auricular branches
and posterior belly of the
digastric muscle

cervical branches

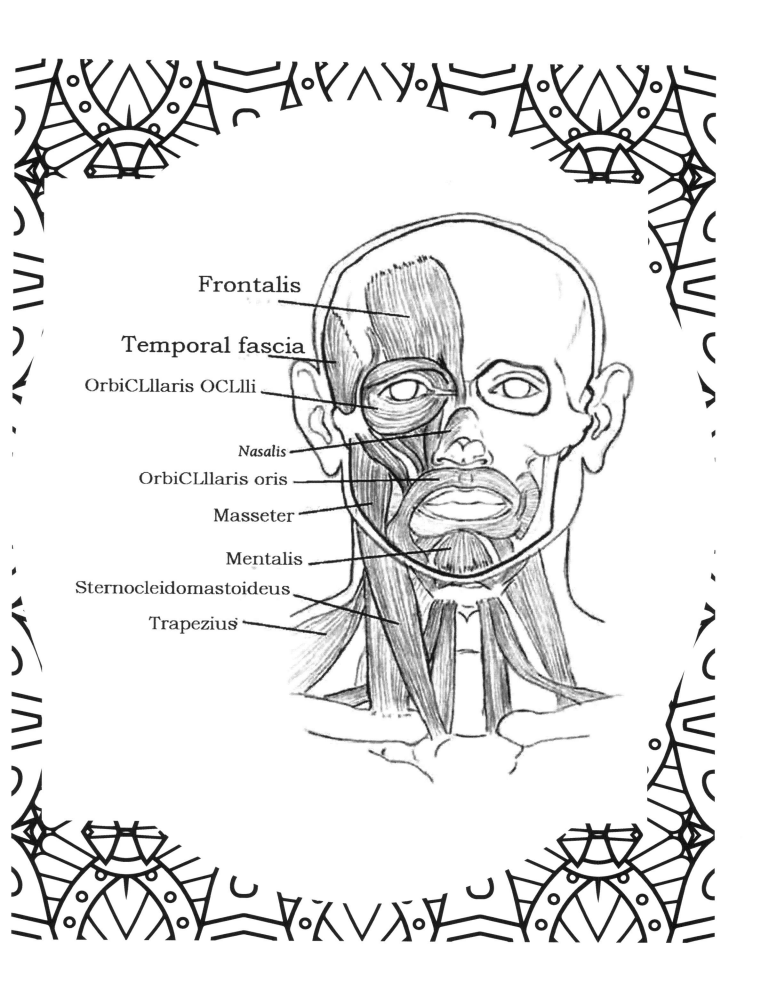

Frontalis

Temporal fascia

OrbiCLllaris OCLlli

Nasalis

OrbiCLllaris oris

Masseter

Mentalis

Sternocleidomastoideus

Trapezius

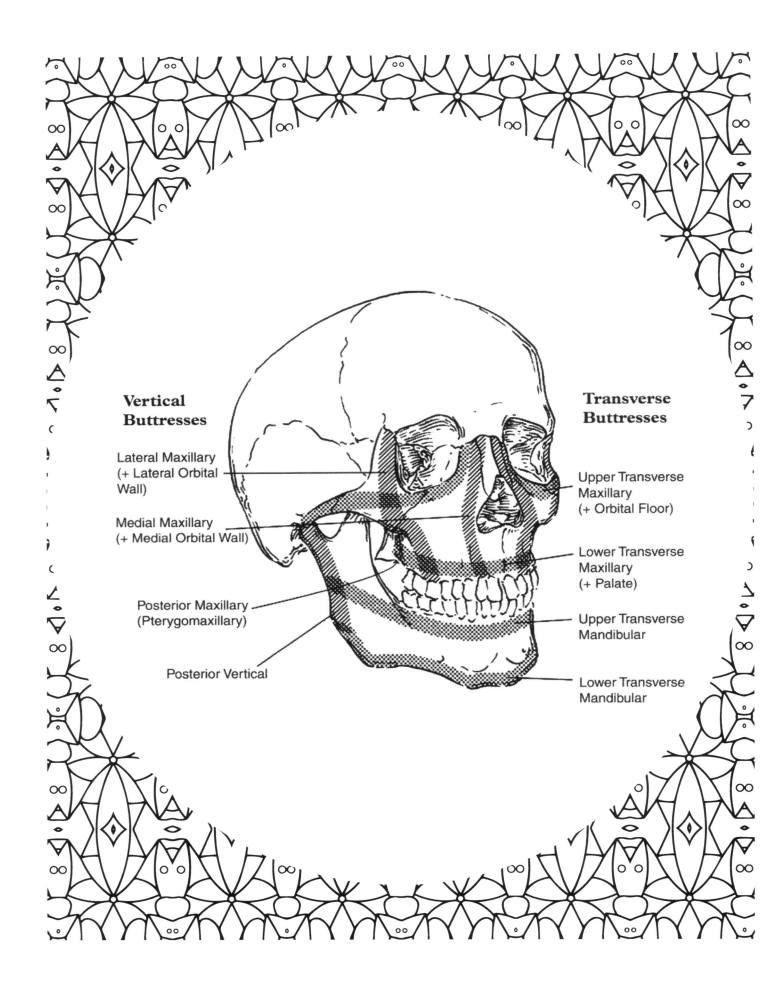

Vertical Buttresses

Lateral Maxillary (+ Lateral Orbital Wall)

Medial Maxillary (+ Medial Orbital Wall)

Posterior Maxillary (Pterygomaxillary)

Posterior Vertical

Transverse Buttresses

Upper Transverse Maxillary (+ Orbital Floor)

Lower Transverse Maxillary (+ Palate)

Upper Transverse Mandibular

Lower Transverse Mandibular

Facial Lifting Effect

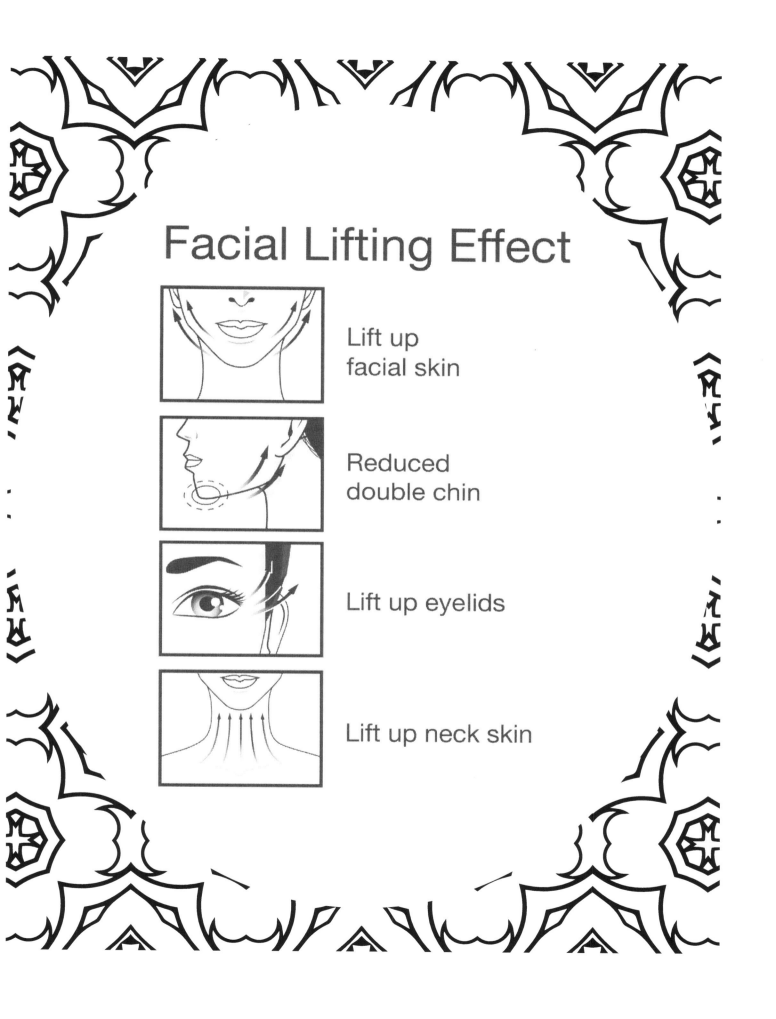

Lift up
facial skin

Reduced
double chin

Lift up eyelids

Lift up neck skin

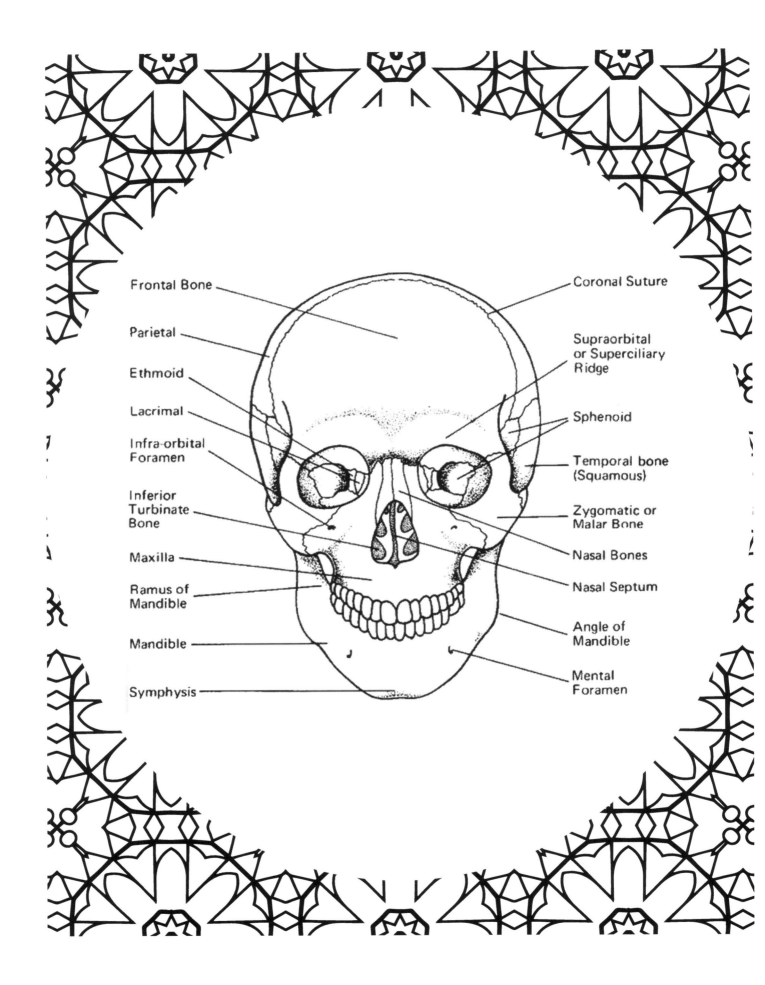

Frontal Bone

Parietal

Ethmoid

Lacrimal

Infra-orbital Foramen

Inferior Turbinate Bone

Maxilla

Ramus of Mandible

Mandible

Symphysis

Coronal Suture

Supraorbital or Superciliary Ridge

Sphenoid

Temporal bone (Squamous)

Zygomatic or Malar Bone

Nasal Bones

Nasal Septum

Angle of Mandible

Mental Foramen

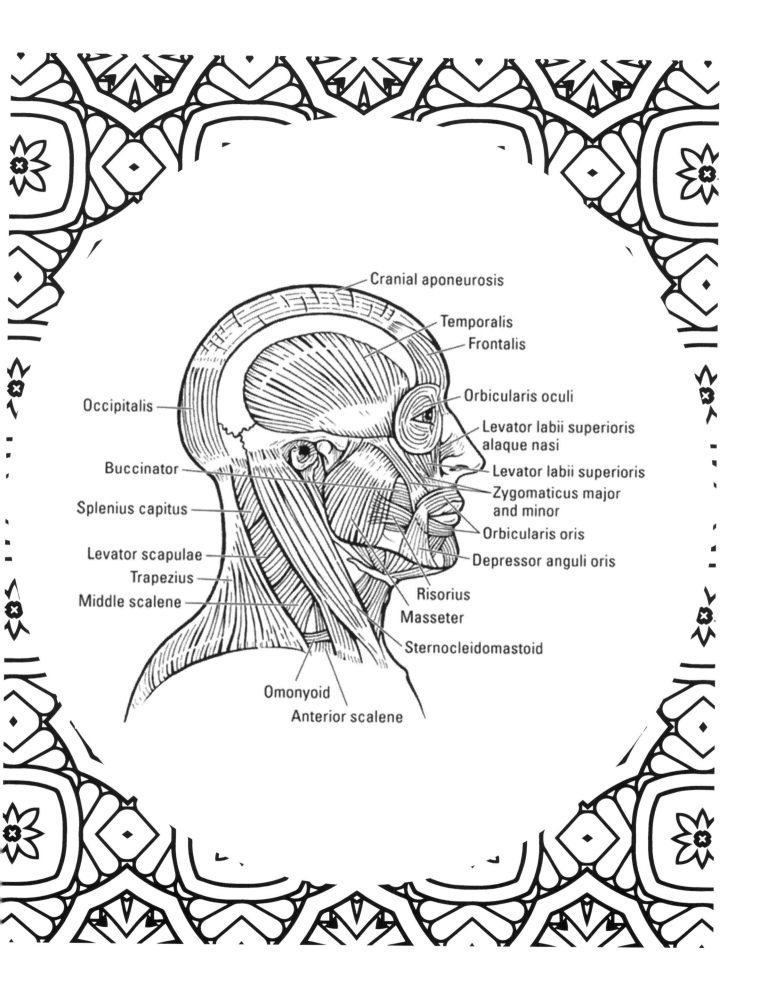

Cranial aponeurosis

Temporalis

Frontalis

Orbicularis oculi

Levator labii superioris alaque nasi

Levator labii superioris

Zygomaticus major and minor

Orbicularis oris

Depressor anguli oris

Occipitalis

Buccinator

Splenius capitus

Levator scapulae

Trapezius

Middle scalene

Risorius

Masseter

Sternocleidomastoid

Omonyoid

Anterior scalene

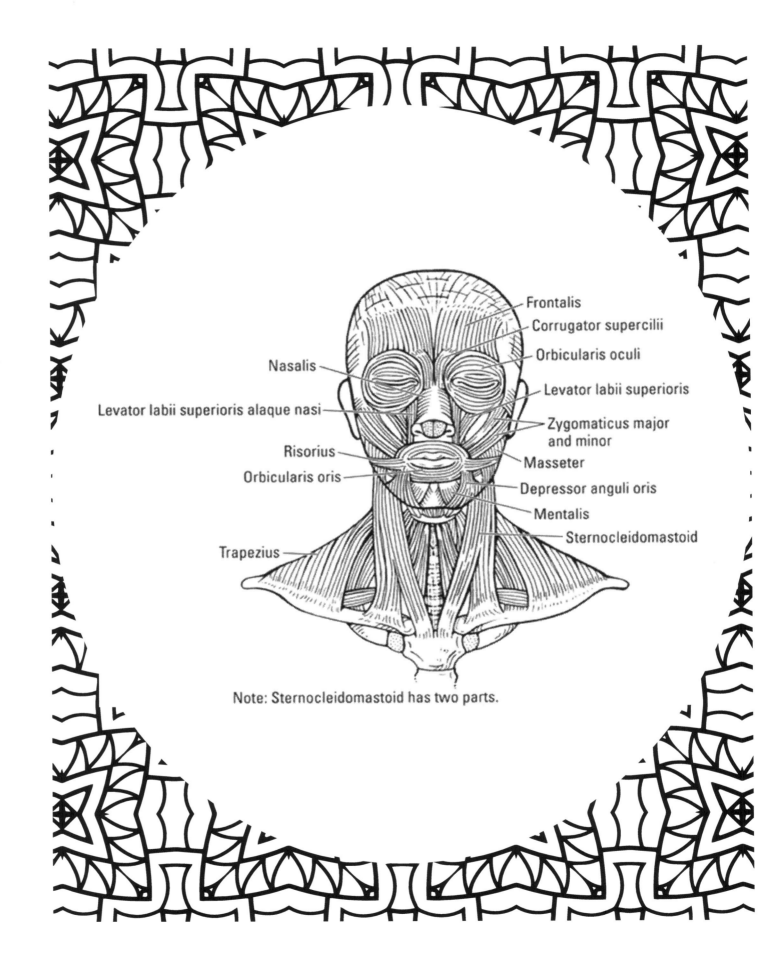

Frontalis

Corrugator supercilii

Orbicularis oculi

Nasalis

Levator labii superioris

Levator labii superioris alaque nasi

Zygomaticus major and minor

Risorius

Masseter

Orbicularis oris

Depressor anguli oris

Mentalis

Sternocleidomastoid

Trapezius

Note: Sternocleidomastoid has two parts.

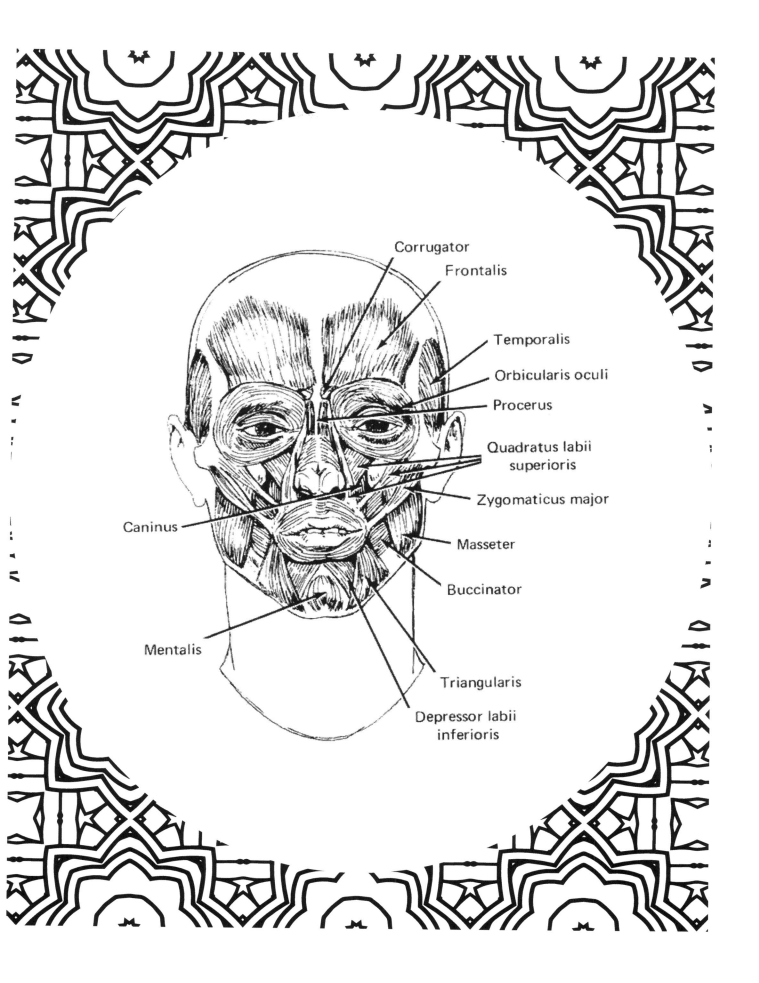

Corrugator

Frontalis

Temporalis

Orbicularis oculi

Procerus

Quadratus labii superioris

Zygomaticus major

Caninus

Masseter

Buccinator

Mentalis

Triangularis

Depressor labii inferioris

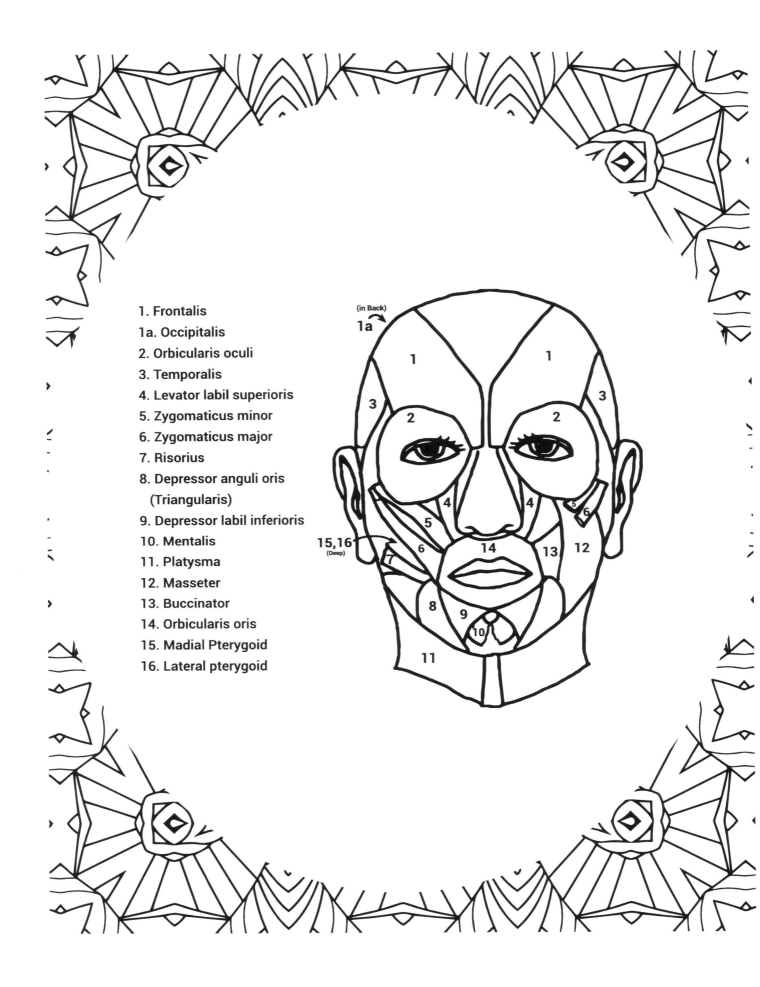

1. Frontalis
1a. Occipitalis
2. Orbicularis oculi
3. Temporalis
4. Levator labil superioris
5. Zygomaticus minor
6. Zygomaticus major
7. Risorius
8. Depressor anguli oris
   (Triangularis)
9. Depressor labil inferioris
10. Mentalis
11. Platysma
12. Masseter
13. Buccinator
14. Orbicularis oris
15. Madial Pterygoid
16. Lateral pterygoid

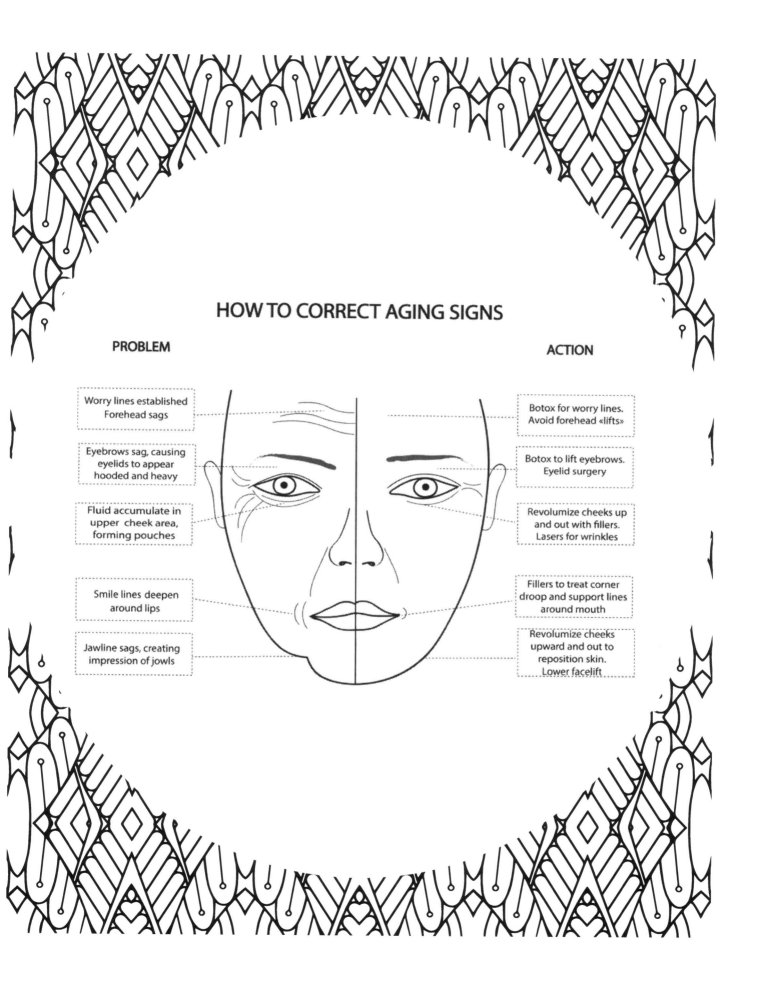

HOW TO CORRECT AGING SIGNS

PROBLEM

ACTION

Worry lines established
Forehead sags

Botox for worry lines.
Avoid forehead «lifts»

Eyebrows sag, causing
eyelids to appear
hooded and heavy

Botox to lift eyebrows.
Eyelid surgery

Fluid accumulate in
upper cheek area,
forming pouches

Revolumize cheeks up
and out with fillers.
Lasers for wrinkles

Smile lines deepen
around lips

Fillers to treat corner
droop and support lines
around mouth

Jawline sags, creating
impression of jowls

Revolumize cheeks
upward and out to
reposition skin.
Lower facelift

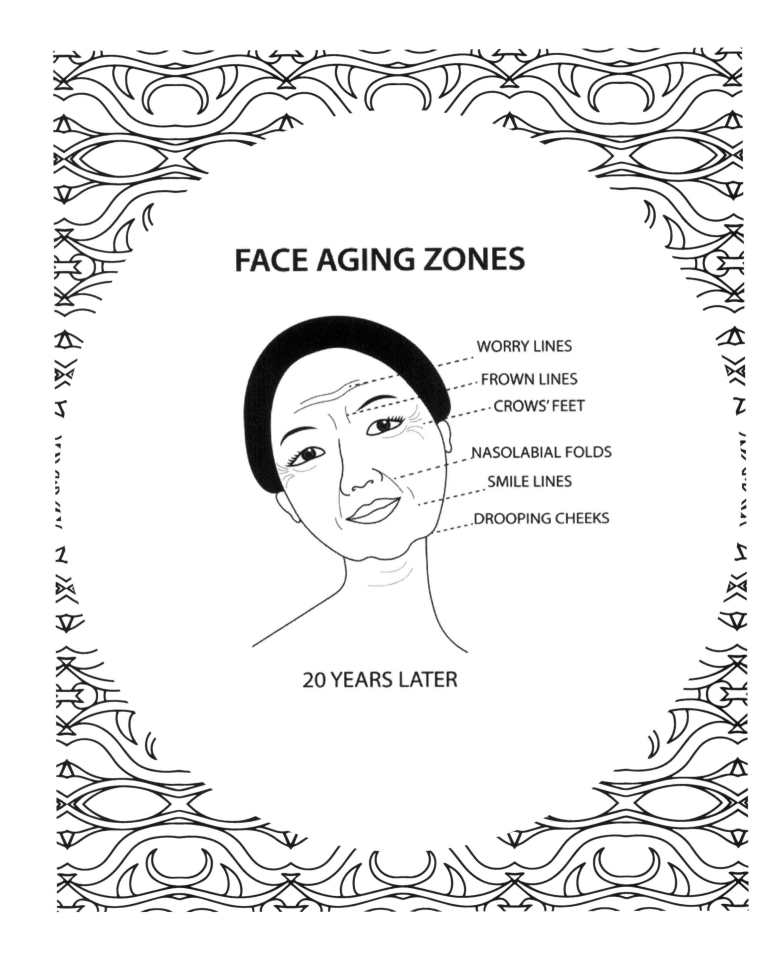

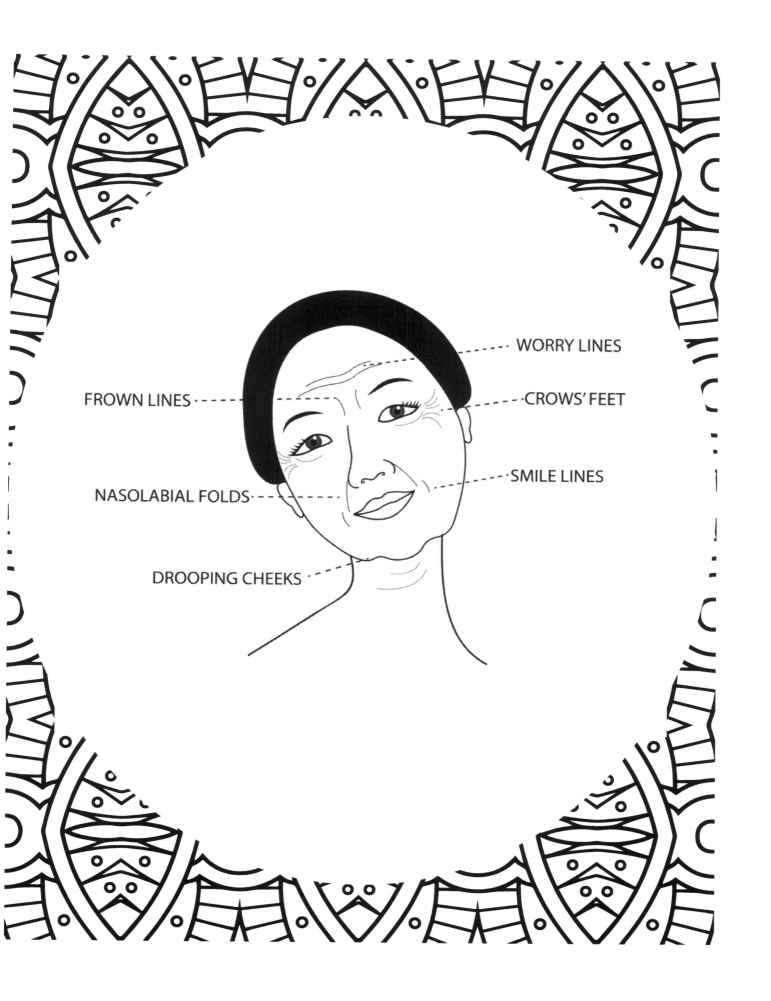

WORRY LINES

FROWN LINES

CROWS' FEET

SMILE LINES

NASOLABIAL FOLDS

DROOPING CHEEKS

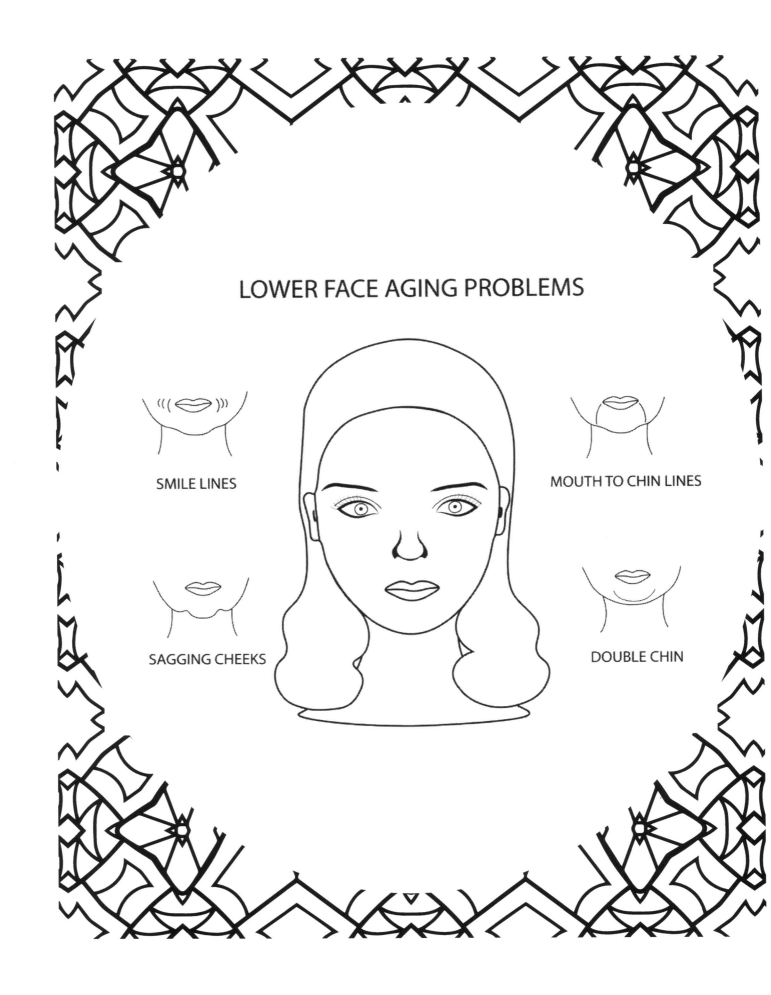

LOWER FACE AGING PROBLEMS

SMILE LINES

MOUTH TO CHIN LINES

SAGGING CHEEKS

DOUBLE CHIN

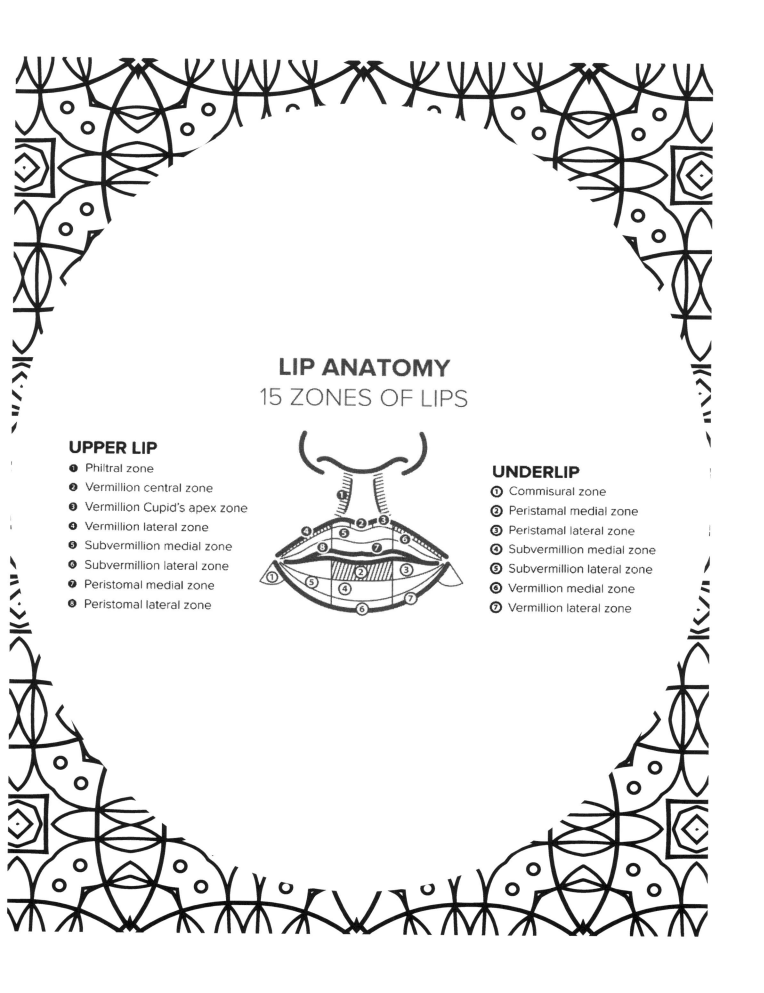

LIP ANATOMY
15 ZONES OF LIPS

UPPER LIP

❶ Philtral zone
❷ Vermillion central zone
❸ Vermillion Cupid's apex zone
❹ Vermillion lateral zone
❺ Subvermillion medial zone
❻ Subvermillion lateral zone
❼ Peristomal medial zone
❽ Peristomal lateral zone

UNDERLIP

① Commisural zone
② Peristamal medial zone
③ Peristamal lateral zone
④ Subvermillion medial zone
⑤ Subvermillion lateral zone
⑥ Vermillion medial zone
⑦ Vermillion lateral zone

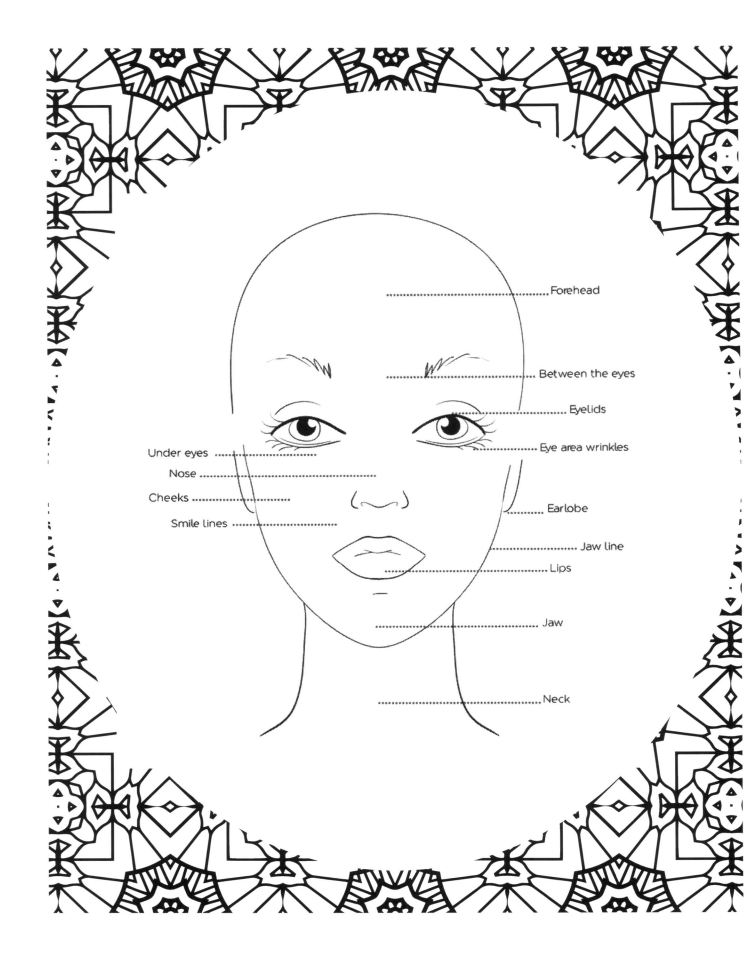

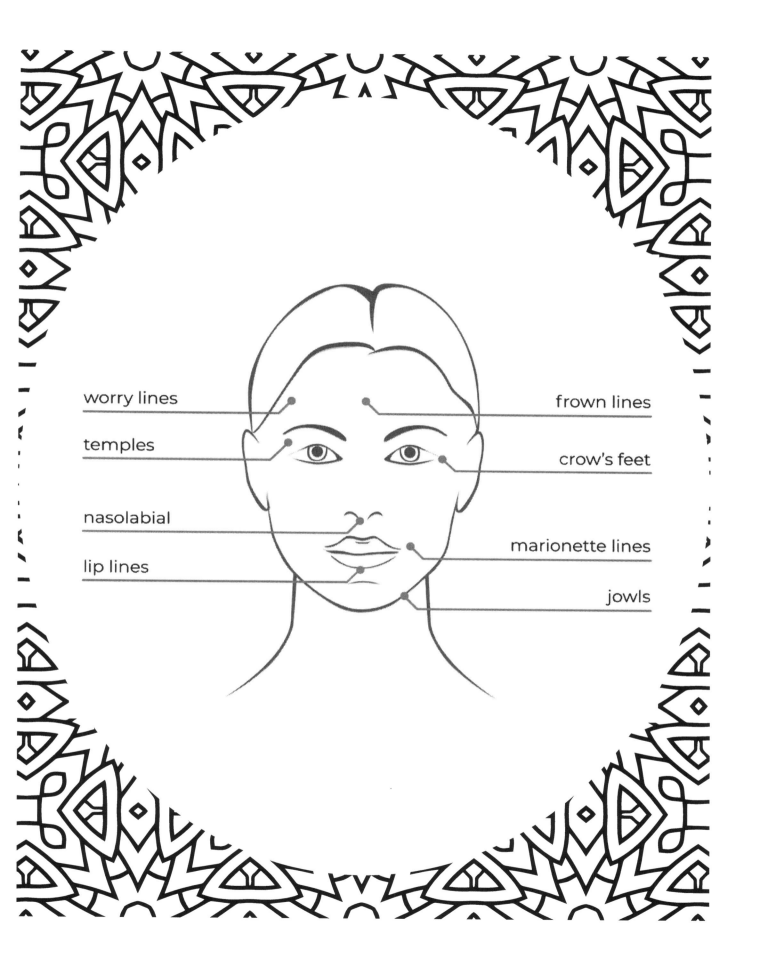

worry lines

temples

nasolabial

lip lines

frown lines

crow's feet

marionette lines

jowls

This Book Belongs To

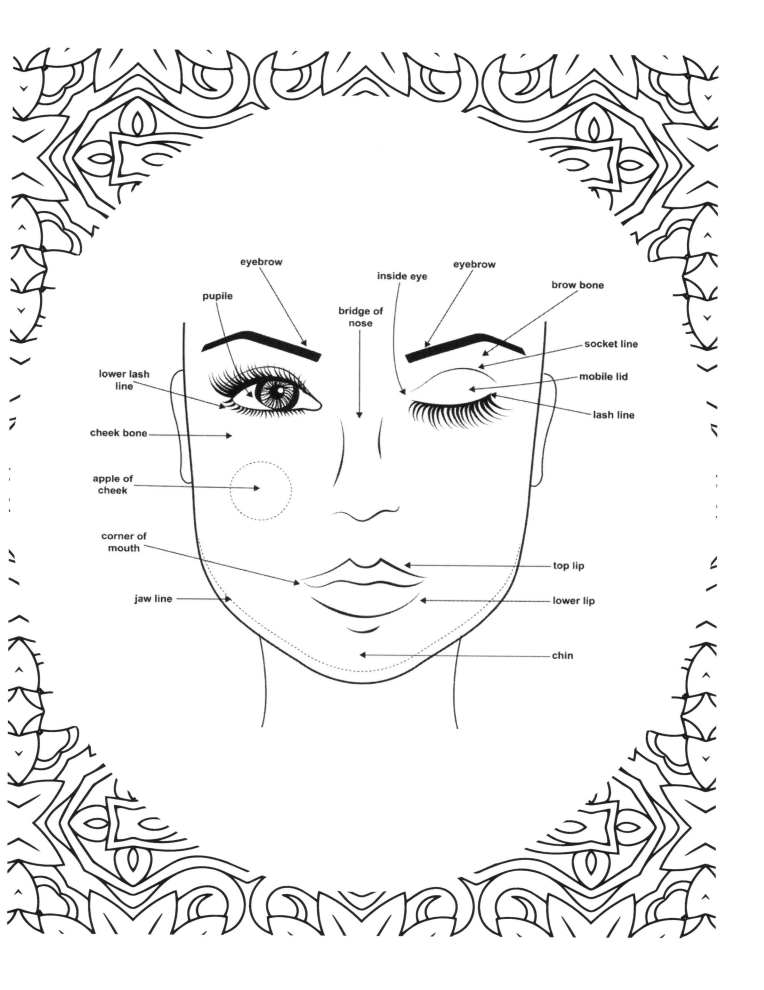

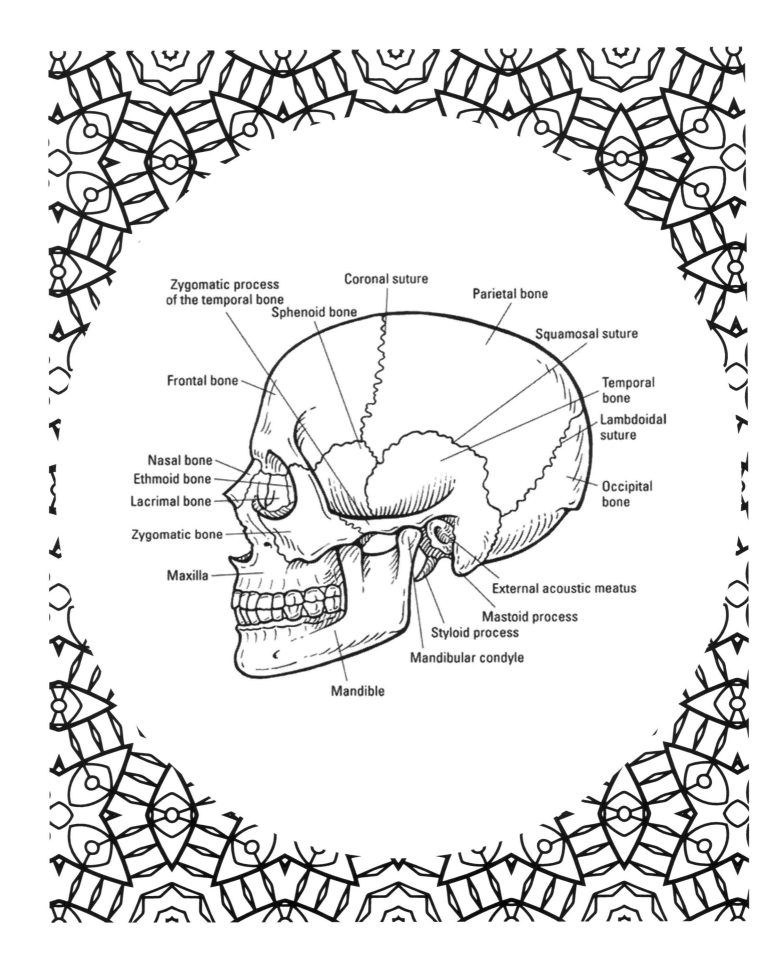

Printed in Great Britain
by Amazon

69093512R00016